T0077623

The Essential Shotokan Series
Companion Workbook

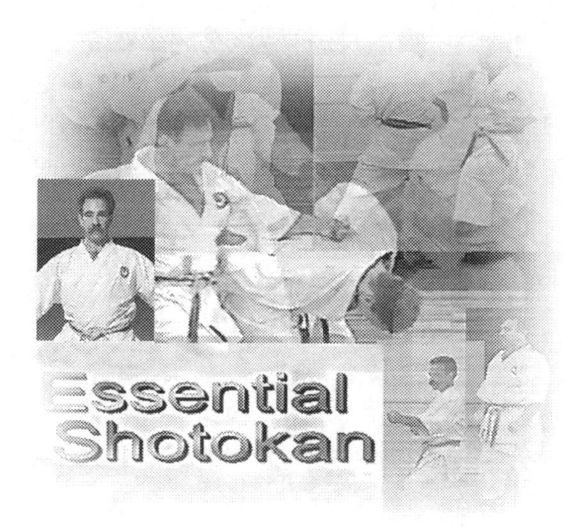

Volume 1:

Principles of Body Dynamics and Stances

by

Edmond Otis, 7th Dan
Chief Instructor & Chairman, American JKA Karate Association
Director of Martial Arts, University of California at Riverside

&

David Gómez, 4th Dan
Senior Instructor, Georgia Karate Academy, Inc.
Associate Instructor, American JKA Karate Association
Adjunct Karate Instructor, Gainesville College Oconee Campus

THE "HOW TO" KARATE SERIES

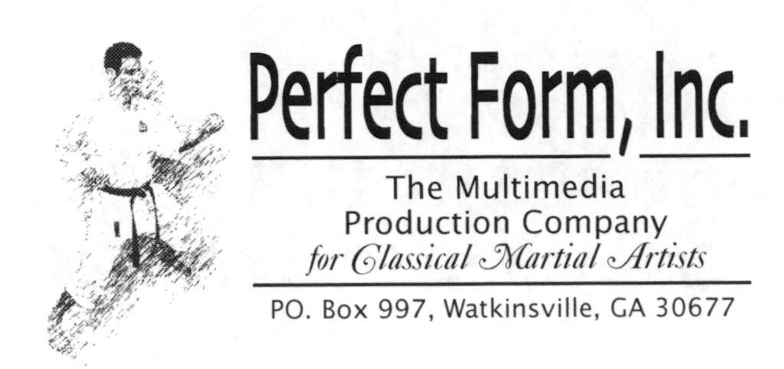

Layout and Design by David Gómez

Warning:

Neither the authors nor the publisher accepts or assumes any responsibility or liability for any personal injuries sustained by anyone as a result of the use or practice of any of the instructions contained in this volume.

This book contains exercises and practice techniques that pertain to karate, self-defense, and combative sparring. Using these techniques and exercises may result in personal injury if not done correctly. In addition, any physical exercise may be physically strenuous, and anyone planning to begin any form of physical training or karate practice is strongly encouraged by the authors to seek medical advice and counsel before beginning. The authors, publisher, and all parties connected to the production of this text accept no responsibility for injuries that may occur through karate training or using the techniques and training practices presented or suggested in this text.

Order this book online at www.trafford.com
or email orders@trafford.com

Most Trafford titles are also available at major online book retailers.

Print information available on the last page.

ISBN: 978-1-4120-4949-8 (sc)

Trafford rev. 11/26/2021

North America & international
toll-free: 844-688-6899 (USA & Canada)
fax: 812 355 4082

Training and practical application outweigh theory, but you have to have a starting place. Set yourself a foundation by consistently training in fundamental technique and principle. Practical application will work its way from there . . .

David Gómez

Table of Contents

DVD/VHS Outline of Contents

IV Stances

1 - Overview (of all stances)

2 - Natural (ready) Stance

- Key Points

3 - Free Stance

- Key Points
- Common Errors
- Review
- Stance in Action

4 - Front Stance

- Key Points
- Common Errors
- Training Method
- Review
- Stance in Action

5 - Back Stance

- Key Points
- Common Errors
- Training Method
- Review
- Stance in Action

6 - Hour Glass Stance

- Key Points
- Common Errors
- Training Method
- Review

7 - Side Stance

- Key Points
- Common Errors
- Training Method
- Review
- Stance in Action

V Also Available in the Essential Shotokan Series

1 - Essential Shotokan Volume 2: Punching and Blocking

2 - Essential Shotokan Volume 3: Kicking and Striking

Available at
www.essential-shotokan.com

Acknowledgments

Randall G. Hassell, Chief Instructor of the American Shotokan Karate Alliance, President of the American JKA Karate Association, a first generation American pioneer of Shotokan karate, a respected writer, editor, and publisher of Tamashii Press, and contributor to numerous books about karate, who in a handful of instances shared time with me outside the dojo and graciously imparted to me anecdotes and first-hand accounts of the early days of Shotokan in the United States, and who graciously gave us permission to use some of his copyrighted materials in this workbook. Some of the line art in this workbook is from *Karate Training Guide, Volume 1: Foundations of Training*, by Randall G. Hassell, published by Focus Publications (www.TamashiiPress.com) . . . thank you!

Mark Groenewold, author and web master of the much acclaimed book and web site of the same name, *Karate The Japanese Way* (www.karatethejapaneseway.com), who currently (2004) lives and trains Shotokan in Kanazawa, Japan, owns and operates UPJ Publications, is an editor and a professor of English. He kindly agreed to edit this workbook for us . . . thank you!

Dedicated To . . .

. . . Vincent Butta *Sensei*, my first Shotokan karate instructor, who set the foundation–molded the core of my Shotokan–and instilled in me a love for traditional karate. To this day, no matter what I learn from all the gifted Shotokan instructors I train with, or have trained with, the "all I do" concerning karate goes back to Butta *Sensei's* dedication to a life of teaching traditional Shotokan karate.

. . . all the Instructors from the AJKA who I have trained with throughout the years as well as all the instructors from various traditional backgrounds and affiliations that have influenced my karate. Every gifted instructor I have trained with has made a "karate imprint," which I will carry forever. This imprint is found in this work. Thank you.

. . . Blaze and Joshua Gómez, my beloved wife and my precious only son. Countless hours I spend doing karate, talking karate, writing karate books, producing educational film/digital media and/or video about karate, traveling to karate camps, clinics, seminars, tournaments, teaching engagements, and not once has Blaze or Jag ever complained. I like karate, but I love them–they give my life meaning. I could not do what I do without their support. Thank you Blaze and Jag. I love you dearly.

David Gómez
Senior Instructor, Georgia Karate Academy, Inc.
Associate Instructor, American JKA Karate Association
Adjunct Karate Instructor, Gainesville College Oconee Campus

Preface

While you are reading and working through this workbook, please remain aware of two points. The first is that the body of the written text in this workbook is a transcription from the narration, demonstrations, and instruction by Edmond Otis found in *Volume 1: Principles of Body Dynamics and Stances* of the *Essential Shotokan* series. The second point is that some of the written material in this workbook was written specifically to interpret or clarify the instruction and demonstrations found throughout this volume. Many concepts, principles, and terms have been incorporated into this workbook as written detail that otherwise might have been missed in the visual presentation of this volume. This workbook is intended as a companion piece to the visual presentation of the *Essential Shotokan* series.

To say that the *Essential Shotokan* series and this accompanying workbook are exhaustive would be an overstatement. The study of traditional Shotokan karate techniques and principles continues to progress from generation to generation, as it should. We do believe, however, that the core essentials of traditional Shotokan karate are represented in the *Essential Shotokan* series, *Volume 1: Principles of Body Dynamics and Stances, Volume 2: Punching and Blocking*, and *Volume 3: Kicking and Striking.* We believe that this workbook is a valuable companion study tool for the beginner, intermediate, or advanced *karateka.* We hope you do, too!

Foreword

Edmond Otis is one of the finest practitioners of JKA-style Shotokan karate in the world, and he personifies a treasure trove of experience and technical excellence at every level of the karate spectrum. He has been a highly successful national and international competitor, and he is known today for his outstanding technique, his innovative teaching methods, and his superb performance as an international referee and judge.

When I first viewed his videotape series, *Essential Shotokan*, I wrote that the tapes were, ". . . the best example I have ever seen of directly relating theory to action. The technique demonstrated is strong, clean, and classic in form."

Now, in collaboration with David Gómez, himself a fine, high-level practitioner of JKA-style Shotokan karate, he has managed to improve on his excellent tapes via the written word.

The *Companion Workbook* to the *Essential Shotokan* series is truly innovative. The instructions are clear and concise, the design and binding are inviting and functional, and the authors skillfully emphasize particularly important points in "Insight" boxes. The ample spaces for notes and the question and answer sections are unique and exceptionally valuable for self-study.

I highly recommend the *Companion Workbook* for the *Essential Shotokan* video and DVD series to anyone who is interested in learning the essentials of Shotokan karate in a logical, progressive, self-paced manner as well as to experienced practitioners who want to review the essential principles of Shotokan.

Both beginners and advanced will benefit greatly from this ingenious workbook.

Randall G. Hassell
Chief Instructor, American Shotokan Karate Alliance
President, American JKA Karate Association

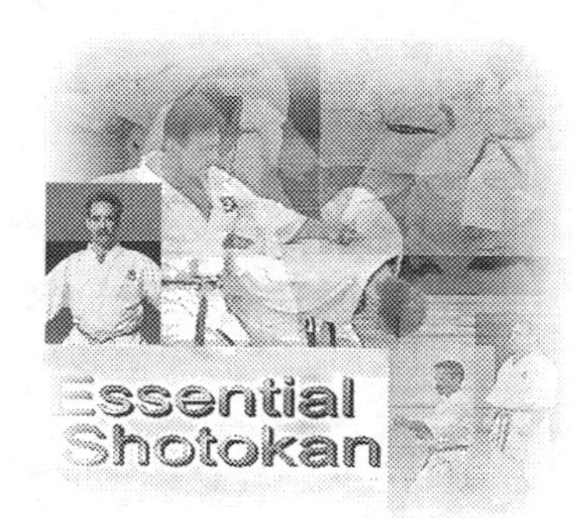

Chapter 1: Introduction

Welcome to the world of Essential Shotokan. The Essential Shotokan Series is intended as a training aid. It presents beginning, intermediate, and advanced applications of Shotokan karate's fundamental techniques. More importantly, it is designed for each technique to be studied in terms of Shotokan's core principles: *focus, body dynamics, stance, breathing, posture,* and *timing.* What makes the Shotokan style of karate so unique and effective is the commitment to studying the relationship between these factors and the techniques themselves.

For the Shotokan stylist, the most advanced technique is frequently the simplest technique. It is defined by its depth, its correctness, and its intensity. In reality, an advanced technique is not what most people think of as a difficult, complex, or intricate set of movements.

Ultimately our goal in training is to sidestep, bypass, or rise above the need for violent conflict. But if this is impossible, we train to develop a level of technical and emotional mastery that allows us to be at our strongest precisely at the moment our opponent is at their weakest.

This volume of Essential Shotokan stands alone, but also serves as one of the three core works in the Essential Shotokan series.

Notes:

Insight to Kick Around

Train to develope a level of technical & emotional mastery.

Notes:

The Essential Shotokan series consists of: *Volume 1, Principles of Body Dynamics and Stances; Volume 2, Punching and Blocking;* and *Volume 3, Kicking and Striking*. We hope you enjoy the Essential Shotokan series and find it of value.

Q and A

1 – The Essential Shotokan series is designed only for advanced karate students.
❑ True
❑ False

2 – The relationship between core principles and technique makes the study of Shotokan unique.
❑ True
❑ False

3 – The ultimate goal in training in karate is to handle a conflict with violence.
❑ True
❑ False

4 – Should karate training develop a level of technical and emotional mastery to be used when an opponent is at their weakest?
❑ Yes
❑ No

Chapter 2: Using Essential Shotokan

Essential Shotokan is a self-paced teaching series designed for the beginner, intermediate, or advanced Shotokan practitioner. These series of volumes are laid out in a practical, easy-to-study, and easy-to-use format, that utilizes two and sometimes three camera angles.

The Format of The Essential Shotokan Series Consists of the Following

Throughout the volumes of the Essential Shotokan series, you will be presented with a series of topics related to Shotokan, such as principles of power, stances, blocking, punching, kicking, and striking. At the beginning of each major topic, a screen will appear, displaying the heading for the material about to be presented, accompanied by a variety of audio markers, usually the sound of a gong. Both the display screen and the audio marker serve as indicators that you are about to view a new major topic in the Essential Shotokan series.

Each major topic presented in the series may be accompanied by sub-topics. Each sub-topic will be identified as:

- Overview
- Key Point
- Common Error
- Training Method

Notes:

Insight to Kick Around
At all levels of experience, self-paced study is not only necessary, it's vital.

Notes:

Sub-topics also will be accompanied by a variety of audio markers, chimes to be exact, to denote sub-topic transitions.

The purpose of the topic and sub-topic display screens is two-fold: first, by dividing this teaching series with visual and audio markers, you will know clearly when you transition from one major topic to another; second, if for example, you wish to view just the topics related to training methods, or just the key points, by simply using the fast forward on your DVD or VCR remote, and keeping your eye out for your topic of interest, you can quickly go to the material you wish to study.

To assist you in finding specific topics, *please refer to the* ***outline of the material covered in this volume*** *located in the enclosed documentation of the Essential Shotokan packaging.*

Remember, the Essential Shotokan series is designed as a tool to be used. But, just like learning to use any tool, it is recommended you have a qualified instructor to assist you as you learn.

Well, it's time to get started! Get your note pad, pencil, the outline that came with your DVD or VHS tape, your DVD or VHS remote, and lets dig in–*Hajime* (means "begin" in Japanese)!

Note

The outline is also found on page "vii" of this companion workbook.

Chapter 3: Principles of Power

Focus Focus Focus

Notes:

Focus–Key Points

By far, one of the most essential aspects and concepts of Shotokan karate is that of *focus,* or concentration of strength. The Shotokan stylist frequently sacrifices fancy or elaborate, complex technique to invest their energy in one or two decisive techniques. We do this by coordinating the reaction and actions of the body with breathing and the technique.

In the study of Shotokan karate, it helps to think of *focus* as a very simple formula: generate as much force as possible in the shortest period of time. We want to deliver that force, as much force as we can, in the shortest possible period of time, into the smallest impact area. To do that, two things are important:

Insight to Kick Around
Focus is the sum total of reaction, body dynamics, breathing, & technique.

Notes:

Insight to Kick Around
Relaxed, but alert, is the key to the shortest "range of time" between no movement and the moment of focus.

Range

By range, we don't literally mean how big our technique is, but instead, how vast an area we have between being as relaxed as possible and as tight as possible when delivering a technique. Range and *focus* meet: our body is soft during the movement and compressed at the end of the movement (technique).

One method Shotokan stylists use to train a soft movement, and to then be compressed at the end of the movement (technique) as an aspect of *focus* and "range" (as defined above), is by "holding" the end of the technique. It is not uncommon during a training session to hear an instructor tell the class, *"Don't move, don't move, and don't move!"* at the end of performing a technique. Then, after a period of not moving/holding the technique in place, students will be told to set up and do the technique again. *The reason we don't move is not that the technique actually takes that long to deliver its force, but to teach the body to recognize the optimal position and relationship of muscles for our body to assume at the moment of impact.*

Combining Body Actions with Breathing

When training, it is important to coordinate the action of the body, whether vibration, rotation, or shifting (which are discussed in greater detail in subsequent chapters), and breathing during the movement, with the actual course of the technique.

Notes:

In every technique, our body moves (vibration, rotation, shifting, etc.), we breathe and we lock at the end of each technique, we relax. Our body moves–we breathe while we move, never holding our breath–we lock, relax . . . and the process repeats. With enough practice, learning to focus this way will yield the techniques that are typical of Shotokan karate.

Q and A

1 – Focus is by far not one of the most essential aspects of Shotokan karate.
- ❑ True
- ❑ False

2 – Focus is a coordination of body reaction, body action, breathing, and technique.
- ❑ True
- ❑ False

3 – A simple formula for focus can be thought of as:
- ❑ To focus, generate as much force as possible, over the longest period of time, into the largest impact area.
- ❑ To focus, generate as much force as possible, over the shortest period of time, into the smallest impact area.

4 – Concerning focus, two things are extremely important:
- ❑ To focus, combine speed and the overall quality of the technique.
- ❑ Combine range and body actions with breathing.

Notes:

5 – It can be said:
- ❑ Moving quickly from one technique to another without interruption will improve the range of focus.
- ❑ One method employed to train a soft movement, to then be compressed at the end of a movement (technique) as an aspect of focus and range, is by holding the end of the technique.

6 – Coordinating body actions with breathing is not as important as muscular strength.
- ❑ True
- ❑ False

Notes:

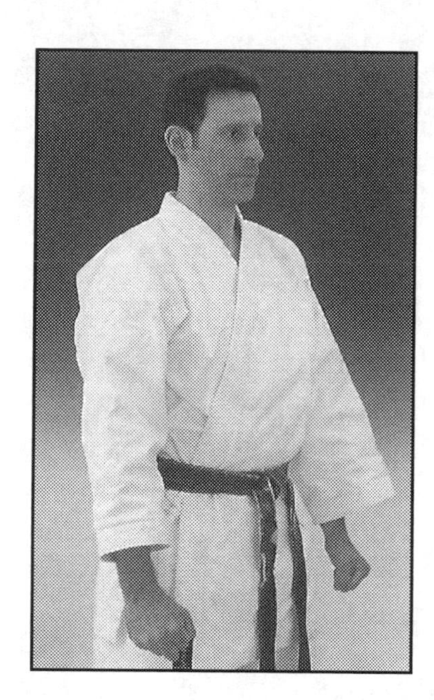

Posture–Key Points

Good posture is essential to the application and performance of all karate-do techniques. Correct posture allows us to move, set, and wait with poise so we can react.

The six key principles for correct posture are:

1-stand with a natural, elongated and straight spine

2-the chin position is pulled back; align the rear of the neck with the spine, chin not protruding over the chest, or "nose-up" exposing the neck

3-keep the shoulders down, resting on the body–no tension in the shoulders or neck

4-maintain stomach and hip tension–tighten the buttocks a little so the hip is engaged with the body center

Insight to Kick Around
Proper posture aligns the body for a maximum transfer of "body dynamics–power".

Notes:

Insight to Kick Around
The six proper posture principles are the key to "correct" stances.

5- relax the body so the muscles remain soft and fluid

6- body weight positioning–push the hips slightly forward so the weight of the body is on the balls of your feet, but keep your heels down on the floor–this will give the body a feeling of readiness and the ability to move quickly

These posture principles apply to all stances–basic, formal, and free. Examples of posture in these stances are demonstrated at the end of "Posture: Key points" on the Essential Shotokan DVD or VHS tape (see outline).

Notes:

Q and A

1 – Correct posture allows us to:
- ❑ relax and sleep
- ❑ move, set, and wait with poise so we can react

2 – One of the six key principles of correct posture is:
- ❑ Keep the body tense at all times.
- ❑ Keep the shoulders down, resting on the body, with no tension.

3 – For correct posture, the body weight position should allow for the heels to be off the floor at all times.
- ❑ True
- ❑ False

Notes:

Insight to Kick Around
The six body actions are not solely used for karate. Body actions develop and transfer power in many activities, i.e., bowling, chopping wood, and swinging a golf club.

Six Body Actions–Overview

There are six primary types of body actions:

1- *Vibration:* This type of body action is the quickest and most immediate. Vibration is accomplished by moving the body's center mass and the hips from left to right (or right to left) in a quick, vibrating fashion.

2- *Body Rotation (hip rotation):* This type of body action is accomplished by rotating the hips and torso from one position to another, using the spine as an axis.

3- *Body Shifting:* Stepping–either forward, back, left or right–or sliding into position.

4- *Body Dropping (Drop Weight):* A simple body action accomplished by lowering the weight of the body by bending the knees and dropping the torso down.

5- *Body Lifting (Lift Weight):* Raising the body weight by using the strength in the legs to lift the body up.

6- *Pendulum Action:* Primarily used in kicking, a pendulum action is a swinging body action where the axis of the hips stays the same, yet the hips lift in place.

Notes:

Q and A

1 – Which is not a body action?
- ❑ muscular strength
- ❑ pendulum action

2 – Pendulum action is primarily used in blocking.
- ❑ True
- ❑ False

3 – Body shifting is done by rotation of the hips.
- ❑ True
- ❑ False

4 – Of all the body actions, vibration is the slowest and least immediate.
- ❑ True
- ❑ False

Notes:

Insight to Kick Around
Even a light object such as a towel can have "heavy" impact if it is snapped back sharply!

Body Vibration–Key Points

The first body action, *body vibration*, is natural to anyone who has ever snapped a towel. To get a good snap, less emphasis is made on the arm and more is placed on the hip, creating a sharp "snap-back".

Two simple examples where *body vibration* (the *action of the body*) is seen in karate are in *straight punch*, from natural stance, and *back fist strike*. In each action during the movement, the body creates the momentum. This momentum transfers to the technique–the straight punch or back fist strike.

Close Up and Review

View the close up and review of *body vibration* as demonstrated on the Essential Shotokan DVD or VHS tape.

NOTE:

Body vibration is initiated from the center mass of the body in a quick, snapping action.

Principle in Action

View the principle of *body vibration* "in action" on the Essential Shotokan DVD or VHS tape.

NOTE:

Body vibration can be accomplished while the body is in motion, without the requirement of a stationary stance/position.

Notes:

Q and A

1 – In body vibration, less emphasis is placed on the hip, and more is placed on the arm.
❑ True
❑ False

2 – Momentum does not play a role in body vibration.
❑ True
❑ False

3 – Body vibration works best with a slow hip snap.
❑ True
❑ False

Notes:

Body/Hip Rotation Key Points

The principle of *body/hip rotation* is used every time something is hit in a way that turns the body. Common examples are swinging a stick, bat, or golf club.

Additionally, there is *reverse reaction rotation.* An example of *reverse reaction rotation* is the motion the hip and body utilize in hitting a tennis ball with a backhand.

Body/hip rotation and *reverse reaction rotation* are seen in numerous karate applications, but a simple example would be reverse punch and lower/downward block.

Close Up and Review

View the close up and review of the *Body/Hip Rotation* section of the Essential Shotokan DVD or VHS tape.

NOTE:

Body/hip rotation pivots the torso, starting where the belly button/torso (from shoulders to pelvic area) is at a 45° angle to a target, until the belly button/torso is no longer at a 45° angle, but is directly facing the target. This also is known as a front-facing hip or squaring the body. The *body/hip rotation* is done quickly and smoothly, focusing the body at the front-facing hip position.

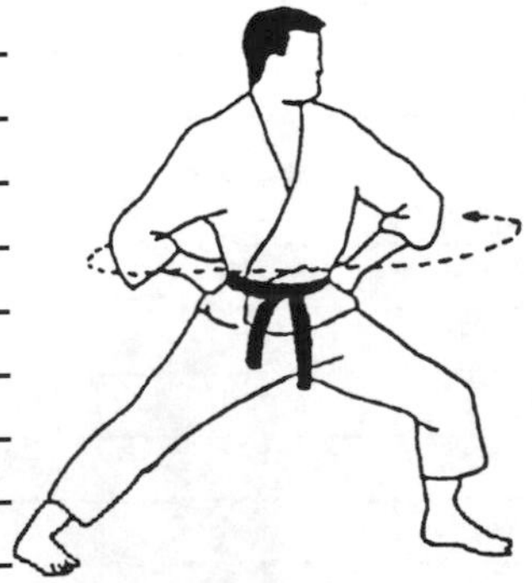

Reverse reaction rotation starts from a front-facing hip position, with the belly button fully facing the target (a square body). Execute the *reverse reaction rotation* with a quick and smooth rotation of

Body/hip rotation ***pivots the torso.***

the torso/hips to a 45° angle relative to the target. Focus the body at the 45° finishing position.

Principle in Action

View the principle of *body/hip rotation* "in action" on the Essential Shotokan DVD or VHS tape.

NOTE:

Smooth and quick *body/hip rotation* is used to execute the defensive blocks and counter punches against the attacker.

Q and A

1 – Body/hip rotation is not used in anything other than karate techniques.
❑ True
❑ False

2 – Reverse reaction rotation is a type of body/hip rotation.
❑ True
❑ False

3 – Body/hip rotation only rotates the hips, leaving the upper part of the torso unmoved.
❑ True
❑ False

4 – A key point in the rotation principle is the similarity to swinging the body with a bat in your hands to hit a baseball.
❑ True
❑ False

Notes:

Insight to Kick Around

Body/hip rotation works best with a smooth movement of the hips; jagged, erratic, or partial rotation minimizes the development and transfer of power.

Notes:

Body Shifting–Key Points

Shifting is a natural body action in which we make power and momentum by moving the body from point "A" to point "B". Anytime you bump or knock into someone, you do *(body) shifting*. If you move your body in a way that displaces another (body), you have done *(body) shifting*.

Examples of body shifting are seen in Oi-tsuki (straight punch or *pursuit attack*) from a natural stance to forward stance, or from natural stance to side stance with an elbow strike (see Body Shifting–Key Points on the DVD or VHS tape for these examples) with either a stepping body action or sliding body action.

Close Up and Review

View the close up and review of the *body shifting* section of the Essential Shotokan DVD or VHS tape.

NOTE:

Body shifting can be performed by stepping (forward, back, left or right) or by sliding the body (in any direction).

Principle in Action

Watch the principle, *body shifting,* "in action" on the Essential Shotokan DVD or VHS tape.

NOTE:

The defensive person starts from an open, natural stance, *shifts* to the rear *by stepping back* into a side stance, *slide shifts* forward in side stance–simultaneously attacking

Notes:

with an elbow strike–then *step shifts* his front foot into a front stance while executing a hammer fist strike.

Q and A

1 – Body shifting creates power by keeping the body still; momentum is not needed.
❑ True
❑ False

2 – An example of body shifting is displacing another person's stance by bumping into them.
❑ True
❑ False

3 – Stepping or sliding the body forward, back, left, or right are both methods of body shifting.
❑ True
❑ False

4 – Body shifting generates power and momentum for striking and punching.
❑ True
❑ False

Insight to Kick Around
Body shifting is accomplished by moving the core center of the body by stepping, sliding, or turning in any direction.

Notes:

Body Dropping–Key Points

Body Dropping is a body action that creates power by dropping the center of the body. An example of this can be seen if you watch someone chopping wood. To chop the wood, the ax is raised above the head and then swung down, simultaneously dropping the body weight with a slight bend of the knees.

An example of *body dropping* in a karate technique can be seen after sweeping an opponent off their feet: we punch down, simultaneously dropping the center of the body by bending the knees. Another example of *body dropping* is elbow strike by *body dropping* from a natural stance to a side stance into a target directly to your front (see these examples on the DVD or VHS tape in the Body Dropping–Key Points section).

Close Up and Review

View the close up and review in the Body Dropping section of the Essential Shotokan DVD or VHS tape.

NOTE:

Body dropping is performed by sharply bending the knees without letting the hips or buttocks bend to the rear. Also note the breathing: exhaling during *body dropping* assists in making the body denser and heavier at the moment of focus.

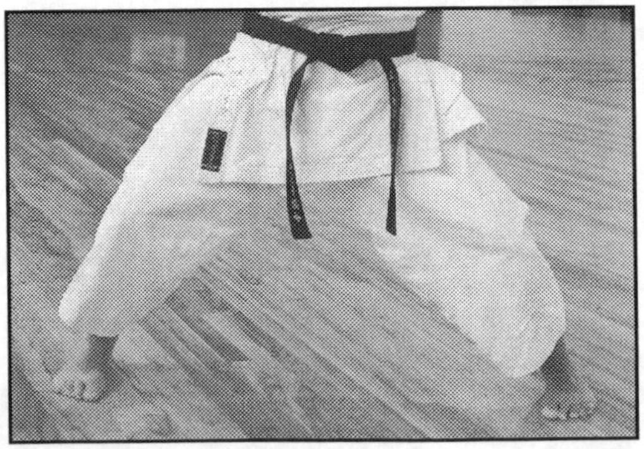

Side stance must have proper posture and uses the principles of body dropping.

Notes:

Principle in Action

Watch the principle, *body dropping,* "in action" on the Essential Shotokan DVD or VHS tape.

NOTE:

Body dropping is done quickly while exhaling and delivering a punch or strike by bending the knees. *Body dropping* does not protrude or misalign the body center, hips, or lower back (away from the target surface).

Q and A

1 – Chopping wood utilizes the principle of body dropping.
❑ True
❑ False

2 – Pushing the body center away from the target and bending fully at the waist is a correct description of the body action known as *body dropping*.
❑ True
❑ False

3 – You should not bend your knees when attempting the body dropping principle.
❑ True
❑ False

4 – It is best to inhale when using the body dropping principle.
❑ True
❑ False

Insight to Kick Around
Drop the body weight, from the core center, with proper posture!

Notes:

Body Raising–Key Points

B*ody raising* is the body action also known as *raising power, body lift, or lift weight.* Power comes from using the legs to raise the body from a low position to a high position.

A simple example of *raising power* is clearly illustrated by squatting down to pick up an object from the floor. Squat down low to the ground and drive up (raise up) the body using the legs (muscles), not the back muscles.

Karate technique examples of the body action principle *body raising* can be seen in rising elbow attack, upper x-block (as a block or strike), and rising block (as a block or strike).

The main point of *body lifting* is to remain low and drive the body up into the attack.

Close Up and Review

View the close up and review in the Body Raising section of the Essential Shotokan DVD or VHS tape.

NOTE:

Body lifting (raising power, body raising, or lift weight) from a low position to a high position is done quickly and smoothly, using the legs to drive the body behind the technique. Exhale during the *body lift*–don't hold your breath.

Principle in Action

Watch the principle, *body raising,* "in action" on the Essential Shotokan DVD or VHS tape.

NOTE:

The rising elbow attack is quickly and sharply executed with the mass of the body creating *raising power.*

Q and A

1 – Body lifting is best done with the muscles of the back.
- ❑ True
- ❑ False

2 – Body lifting drives the body from a low position up into the attack.
- ❑ True
- ❑ False

3 – A good example of body lifting is:
- ❑ keep the knees straight, and bend at the waist to pick up an object from the floor
- ❑ squat down low to the ground, and drive up (raise up) the body using the legs (muscles)

4 – It is best to hold your breath when using the principle of lift weight.
- ❑ True
- ❑ False

Notes:

Insight to Kick Around
Raise the body weight from the core center with the leg muscles–don't bend your back!

Notes:

Pendulum Action Key Points

Pendulum action, or *swinging action*, is usually used in a close distance technique, when you don't have time (or the distance) for a large body action. Basically, the central axis of the hips stays in place, but the *hips rotate up. This is a small body action.*

Examples of pendulum action in karate techniques can be seen in front snap kick and knee attacks. Power is created in the attack by rotating the hips up *into* the front snap kick or the knee.

Close Up and Review

View the close up and review in the Pendulum Action section of the Essential Shotokan DVD or VHS tape.

NOTE:

The *knee is raised* fully over the level of the waist. Then the body action/*pendulum action* rotates the hips up to create power.

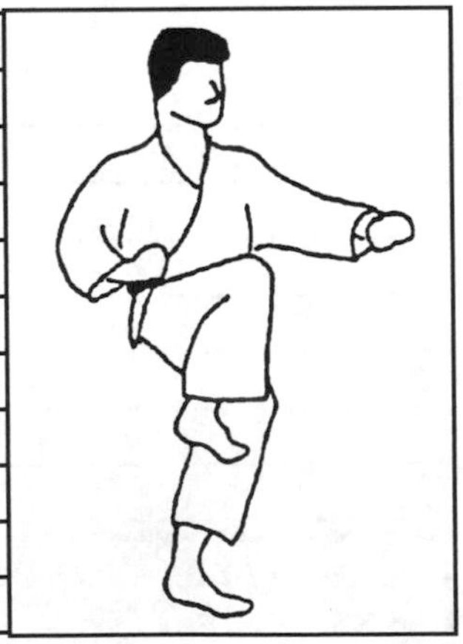

Principle in Action

Watch the principle, *pendulum action,* "in action" on the Essential Shotokan DVD or VHS tape.

NOTE:

In this sequence, the counter attacker's front kicking foot is close to his desired target. His front foot does not have the time or the distance for a large body action; instead, he uses the body action principle, *pendulum action*. By simply *raising the knee* of the kicking leg toward his target,

During a front snap kick first raise the knee fully over the waist, then rotate the hips using a pendulum action.

and then quickly and smoothly rotating his hips upward and into the target (*this is the body action–pendulum action*) with a front snap kick, his kick is highly effective and has much power.

Notes:

Q and A

1 – Pendulum action ideally is used when you are extremely far from your target.
❑ True
❑ False

2 – Pendulum action is a small body action.
❑ True
❑ False

3 – The central axis of the hips rotates in place during pendulum action.
❑ True
❑ False

4 – Pendulum action drives the impact of the kicking foot or knee.
❑ True
❑ False

Insight to Kick Around
Pendulum action is used when you don't have the time or the distance for a large body action.

Notes:

Insight to Kick Around
Proper breathing fully fills the lower part of the lungs first. "Shallow" breathing causes hyperventilation and hinders the technique and focus.

Breathing–Key Points

Proper breathing *coordinates the body to make power for an attack and to protect us if we are hit.* It is important to time the breathing with the technique. In a technique such as straight punch, exhale while performing the technique, and coordinate exhalation to terminate at the moment of focus. Additionally, to assist the body in absorbing an incoming technique, coordinate exhalation to focus at the moment of impact.

The lesson of breathing learned in *taikyoku shodan* (a series of prearranged movements and techniques called *kata,* designed not only to teach breathing but also the use of body dynamics, rhythm, and timing, among other things, that are considered a formal exercise) set the foundation for the breathing lesson taught in the more advanced kata, *heian nidan*.

In the first kata, *taikyoku shodan,* breathing/exhalation is performed once per every technique. In the second kata, *heian nidan,* one breath allows us to perform more than one technique and change the timing. The change of timing allows for three focal compressions during the one breath. An example of this type of breathing can be seen in the Breathing–Key Point(s) section on the Essential Shotokan DVD or VHS tape.

Notes:

Q and A

1 – Breathing during a technique is *only* to prevent you from passing out.
- ❑ True
- ❑ False

2 – What is most important in bringing the breathing and the technique together?
- ❑ timing
- ❑ squeezing the muscles slowly

3 – Breathing (exhaling) plays a role in protecting me by helping to absorb an incoming technique at the point of impact.
- ❑ True
- ❑ False

4 – *Heian nidan* teaches you to exhale once during every technique without multiple focal compressions.
- ❑ True
- ❑ False

5 – Two types of breathing have been discussed: First, one breath per technique; second, one breath with multiple techniques and multiple focal compressions.
- ❑ True
- ❑ False

Notes:

Insight to Kick Around
Timing is a fundamental concept employed for sparring or self-defense tactics.

Timing–Key Points

The most fundamental way to think of timing has to do with addressing an opponent's attack in one of three ways. We can either counter attack ***after*** an opponent's attack–***after*** blocking; we can move with our opponent and counter attack ***during*** the opponent's attack; or we can sense and initiate, advancing upon an opponent fractions of a second ***before*** an opponent's attack.

View the three examples of timing, *after, during, and before* an attack, in the Timing–Key Point(s) section of the Essential Shotokan DVD or VHS tape.

NOTE:
Regarding *the right* ***time*** *to respond to an attack,* the examples just viewed employ the three basic methods of timing:

- after the opponent's attack, after blocking
- during the opponent's attack
- before the opponent's attack

In a general sense, each method of counter attacking–*after, during, or before* an opponent's attack–involves ***how much time*** you have to respond. This is also known as ***catching the timing***. If you're caught off guard ***without enough time*** to respond, making it impossible to counter attack immediately, you counter attack ***after*** blocking. If, however, you're not caught off guard or too late, you ***may have enough time*** to respond with a simultaneous counter response/attack ***during*** the

Notes:

opponent's attack. Lastly, in the best instance, sensing an opponent's impending offensive movement ***allows you the time*** to initiate a counter attack ***before*** an opponent's attack. ***How much time*** you have to respond with a counter attack plays a major role in ***catching the timing after***, ***during***, or ***before*** an opponent's attack.

Rhythm Timing & Reaction Timing–Overview

An alternative way to look at timing has to do with the relationship between *rhythm timing* and *reaction timing*:

- *Rhythm timing* takes into account the movement of your opponent.
- *Reaction timing* has to do with catching your opponent by surprise.

Two examples of *rhythm and reaction timing*, one for offense and one for defense (view these examples on the Essential Shotokan DVD or VHS tape in the Rhythm Timing and Reaction Timing section):

Rhythm Timing Defensively

Rhythm timing defensively allows for use of an opponent's timing/*body movement* and attacking technique to create a window of opportunity to set up a counter attack. As a person front kicks, use his timing and technique to set up a counter attack.

Reaction Timing Offensively

Reaction timing offensively attacks and catches (strikes) an opponent without giving any indication, announcement, or

Insight to Kick Around
Rhythm and reaction timing are strategic tactics used either offensively or defensively.

Notes:

telegraphing intention of attacking by either closing the distance between you and the opponent or catching the opponent standing still.

Timing that is Sooner, Faster, and Deeper

A third way to consider timing is the relationship between *starting time and distance*. This principle of timing teaches karate students to advance with a technique *sooner*, *faster*, and *deeper* against an opponent.

Consider this simple illustration using front kick: if an attacker advances with a front kick, and if the opponent *escapes at the same speed*, then the attacker will have very little chance of catching the opponent with the front kick. If both the attacker and opponent *start at the same* time, there is very little chance of the attacker catching the opponent. If the attacker kicks and the opponent *retreats the same distance* as the attacker, the attacker has very little chance of catching the opponent. However, if an attacker can *start a little sooner, go a little faster, go a little deeper*, then the attacker can change the opponent's distance and catch the opponent with his front kick.

Principle in Action

Watch the principle of *timing that is sooner, faster, and deeper* "in action" on the Essential Shotokan DVD or VHS tape.

Notes:

NOTE:

With the exception of counter attacking *after* blocking, the "in action" just viewed clearly exemplifies *all the principles of timing*. Clearly illustrated are counter attacking *before* and *during* an opponent's attack, *rhythm* and *reaction* timing, and timing that is *sooner*, *faster*, and *deeper*.

Things to Watch For In Each Attack

- In the first attack: The attacker uses the opponent's rhythm of movement to set up and initiate an attack. The attacker *catches the timing before the opponent's attack* by going *sooner, faster, and deeper* using *rhythm timing*.
- Second attack: The attacker feints a jab to the face, causing the opponent to move. The attacker then uses this movement to *catch the timing* with a front kick *during* the opponent's reaction to the feint by going *sooner, faster, and deeper* using *rhythm timing*.
- Third & fourth attack: The initial attacks are thwarted with *reaction timing* by catching the timing in sensing an attack, but closing the distance *sooner*, *deeper*, and *faster* with a counter attack *before* the opponent's attack.

Insight to Kick Around

Catch timing either after, during, or before an attack, use the rhythm or reaction principle, and do it sooner, faster, and deeper!

Notes:

Q and A

1 – The most fundamental way to think of timing has to do with addressing an opponent's attack.
❑ True
❑ False

2 – Regarding the timing principle *after* (an opponent's attack), you respond with a counter attack after blocking.
❑ True
❑ False

3 – Timing the movement to hit an opponent advancing toward you is called catching the opponent *during* the attack.
❑ True
❑ False

4 – How much time you have to respond to an opponent plays a large role in what type of timing response you employ.
❑ True
❑ False

5 – Rhythm timing has to do with catching your opponent by surprise.
❑ True
❑ False

6 – Reaction timing takes into account the movement of your opponent.
❑ True
❑ False

Notes:

7 – Use of an opponent's body movement and technique to set up a counter attack uses which timing principle?
❑ rhythm timing
❑ reaction timing

8 – Catching an opponent by surprise or standing still employs which timing principle?
❑ rhythm timing
❑ reaction timing

9 – If an opponent escapes at the same time, moves the same distance, and travels at the same speed as the attacker, there is very little chance of the attacker catching the opponent.
❑ True
❑ False

Notes:

Chapter 4: Stances

Notes:

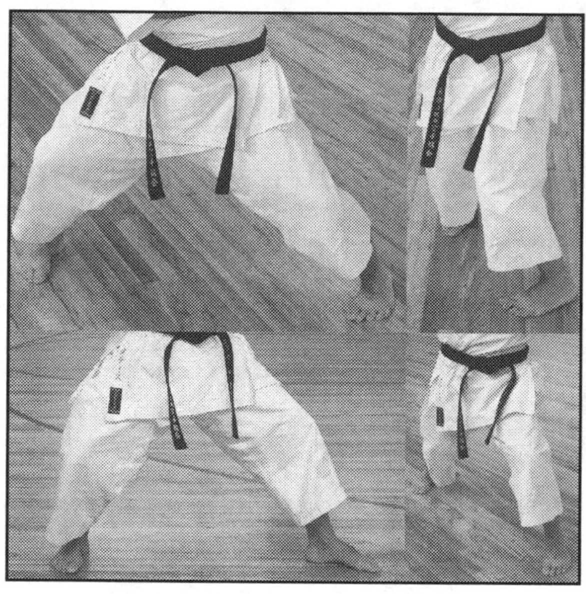

Overview Of All Stances

Many stances are used in karate. This volume of the Essential Shotokan series highlights six of the seven most common stances:

1 - forward stance

2 - side stance

3 - back stance

4 - hour glass stance

5 - free stance

6 - natural stance

7 - cat stance (not covered in this volume)

Insight to Kick Around

Stances are classified as inner or outer tension stances by bowing the knees either towards or away from the body center.

Notes:

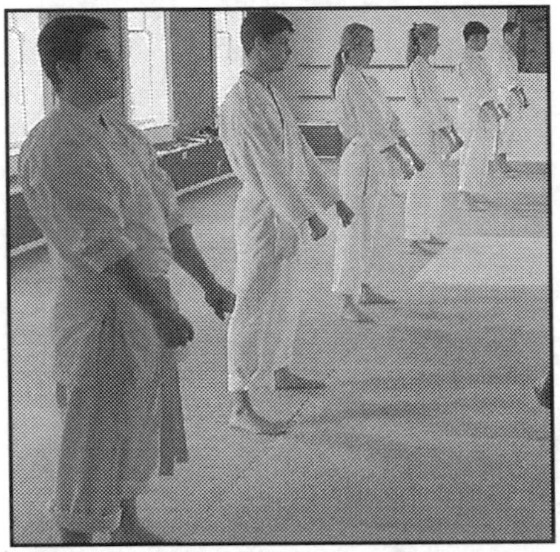

Natural/Ready/*Yoi* Stance–Key Points

Natural stance is a neutral position of readiness. The key points to remember:

- keep your spine straight
- chin back
- shoulders back, down, and relaxed
- the body center is slightly tight
- the tailbone is tucked underneath by gently squeezing the buttocks
- the muscles of the body are relaxed
- the weight of the body is shifted forward on the balls of the feet, helping to engage the hips

Please note, the above listed *natural stance* key points are related to *posture*. A *natural stance* must contain the key elements of good posture; all stances contain the key elements of good posture.

Notes:

Additionally, specifically regarding *natural/ready stance*, the Japanese word, "*yoi*" which literally means, "*Get ready*", is typically used to bring a group of students in training, or contestants of *kumite* (sparring) and/or *kata* (formal exercise drills) to *natural/ready stance.* Technically speaking, calling out "*yoi*" commands a training student and/or a contestant of *kumite* or *kata* to a posture of readiness. One who responds to the "*yoi*" command typically assumes a *natural/ready stance* (position). For this reason, the *natural/ready stance* is also known as the *yoi position*.

Lastly, *natural/ready/yoi stance* is literally a firm "*attention-posture*" stance known as "*Hachiji Tachi*" *(pronounced* as *dachi*, which means stance).

When assuming the *yoi position*, coordinate concentration of mind and body to one focal point. To assume the *yoi* position, the arms go out, up and around (the face), cross the body, and open slightly in front of the hips. The *yoi position* not only prepares the *karateka* (one who does karate), but also indicates to others physical and mental preparation for conflict (sparring) or *kata* (formal training exercise).

NOTE:

View the *natural stance–key points* demonstration on the Essential Shotokan DVD or VHS tape.

Insight to Kick Around

A natural stance is a neutral, yet alert, position of readiness!

Notes:

Q and A

1 – Natural stance, ready stance, and *yoi* position is *Hachiji Tachi.*
❑ True
❑ False

2 – Posture is only important to natural stance when performing *kata.*
❑ True
❑ False

3 – For a good *yoi* position, tighten all your muscles tightly so you can focus your concentration.
❑ True
❑ False

4 – If *yoi* position is done correctly, my opponent will not know I am ready to engage in sparring.
❑ True
❑ False

5 – The command, "*Yoi,*" literally means *ready position.*
❑ True
❑ False

6 – Natural/ready/*yoi* stance coordinates concentration of mind and body.
❑ True
❑ False

Notes:

Free Stance–Key Points

Free stance is a prepared form of natural stance. It is used when the body is uncommitted to any specific action while it is engaged in a conflict or combative role. Free stance is not as long as forward stance (see Front Stance–Key Points, refer to outline) but only three-quarters length of a front stance. The weight of the body is not committed to the front or the back, but rests between the legs. Most of the weight is on the balls of the feet. Tucking the hips underneath the torso ensures moving the body smoothly to the front, side, and back.

Common Errors

Common errors associated with *free stance:*

1- concerning the *lower* body: being too *tense* or *planted* in position, preventing you from being able to move

2- concerning the *upper* body: having the shoulders up (tense) also hinders you from being able to move or respond

3- concerning the *upper and lower* body: being so intent on the opponent in front of you that your face is forward and your hips are back

4- when moving in *free stance:* moving the hands out of time with the movement of the body

Close Up and Review

View the close up and review in the Free Stance section of the Essential Shotokan DVD or VHS tape.

Insight to Kick Around

A natural stance is a neutral, yet alert, position of readiness!

Notes:

NOTE:

Free Stance is not rigid, too low, long, or high as stances go; *free stance* is a comfortable, committed form of natural stance with posture aligned correctly.

Principle in Action

Watch *free stance* "in action" on the Essential Shotokan DVD or VHS tape.

NOTE:

Free Stance allows a *karateka* to move smoothly from stance to stance while executing all types of defensive or offensive counter attacks.

Q and A

1 – Free stance has absolutely nothing in common with natural stance.
❑ True
❑ False

2 – Free stance can be used to engage in a conflict or combative role.
❑ True
❑ False

3 – Free stance is just as long as a forward stance.
❑ True
❑ False

Notes:

4 – Free stance should have the body weight totally committed to the front or to the rear but never smoothly distributed between the legs.
❑ True
❑ False

5 – Free stance generally places most of the weight on the balls of the feet.
❑ True
❑ False

6 – Tucking the hips underneath the torso tightens the lower body and does not allow the body to move smoothly to the front, side, and back.
❑ True
❑ False

7 – Tension in the upper or lower body will prevent a *karateka* from moving in free stance effectively.
❑ True
❑ False

Notes:

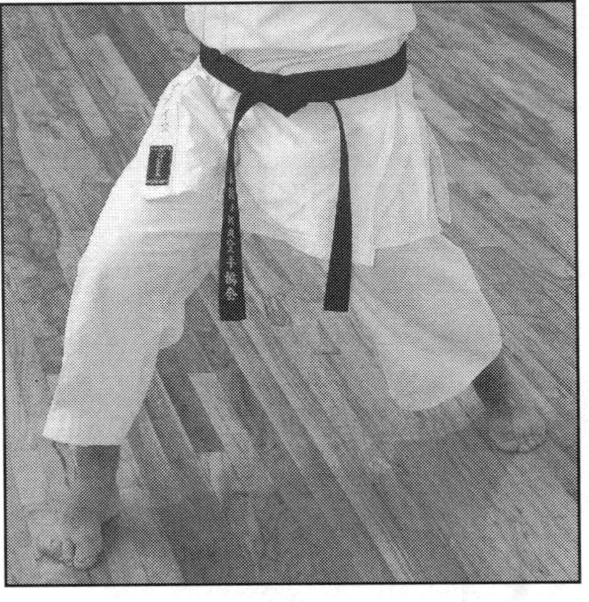

Front Stance–Key Points

Front stance is the most commonly used fundamental karate stance in Shotokan. It is an outside tension stance,which means that the knees push away from the body center in a front stance. The major key points to remember:

- posture remains natural and "correct" (see Principles of Power, Section 2: Posture–Key Points)
- the width of a front stance is as wide apart as the hips
- the length of a front stance is about twice the width of the hips
- the front foot is turned slightly in; the outside edge of the little toe points forward so that the big toe points slightly toward the body center

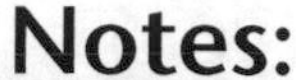

- the back foot is at (about) a 45° angle
- the back foot pushes from the heel–known as driving the heel into the ground–up through the leg, primarily to push the body center and hips forward
- the front foot should "grab" the floor with the toes

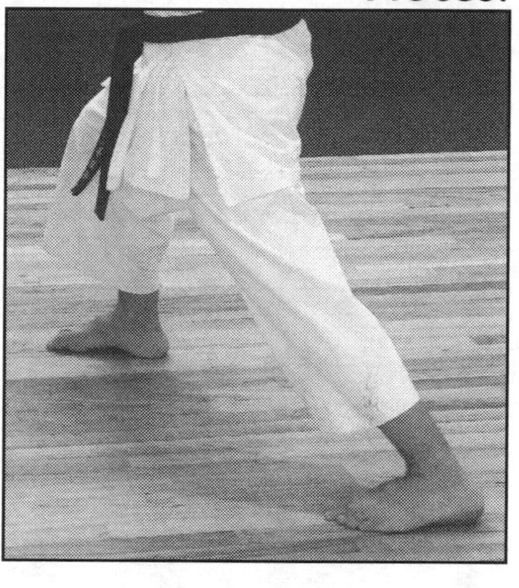

The *most important point* to remember about front stance is that *the back leg does most of the work.* The back leg supplies 60% of the force to the front (body center), allowing the front leg to support the body weight.

Common Errors

Common errors associated with *front stance:*

1 - allowing the hips to go back
- the hips must never go behind the parallel plane of the shoulders in front stance
- the back leg must drive the body center forward

2 - turning the front foot out
- outside tension is ruined (severed) when the front foot is turned out, making it impossible to make force or power in a front stance

3 - placing too much weight on the front leg
- excess weight on the front leg will not allow the proper tension required on the back leg

Forward stance is a *driving* stance; the back leg (via the driving heel) does most of the work; the front leg only supports the body.

Insight to Kick Around
The back leg in a front stance drives 60% of the force to the front by pushing the rear heel into the ground.

Notes:

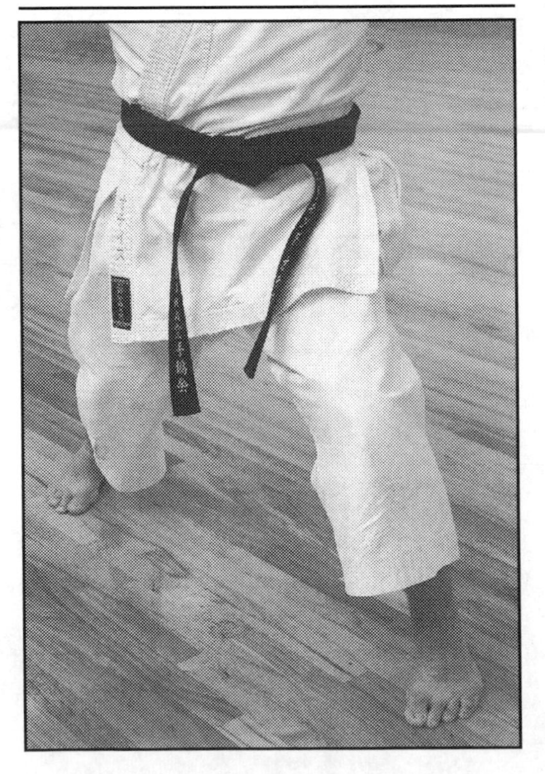

Training Method for Front Stance

Two basic methods to test the strength of front stance:

1- assume a front stance and have someone *exert pressure to the front of the hips*
  - assume a front stance, and have someone push, from the front, at the hips, toward the rear leg

2- test the strength of the back leg
  - assume a front stance, and have someone exert downward pressure against the back of the knee (very carefully and with much caution)
  - a back leg with the proper driving tension will not buckle

Close Up and Review

View the close up and review in the Front Stance section of the Essential Shotokan DVD or VHS tape.

NOTE:

Front stance is as wide as the hips and twice as long. The back leg, starting at the heel, is driving the body center and hips forward, and the back leg is straight. Proper posture is maintained while moving or standing still.

Stance in Action

Watch *front stance* "in action" on the Essential Shotokan DVD or VHS tape.

NOTE:

Front stance maintains the dynamics of outside tension, a driving rear leg, and proper posture while attacking or responding to an attack.

Notes:

Q and A

1 – Front stance has absolutely nothing in common with posture.
❑ True
❑ False

2 – Front stance places most of the weight on the back foot.
❑ True
❑ False

3 – The hips should be driven forward by the tension and extension of the back leg in a front stance.
❑ True
❑ False

4 – The driving force of the back leg starts on the balls of the feet.
❑ True
❑ False

5 – The width of a front stance is as wide as your hips.
❑ True
❑ False

6 – The length of a front stance is about twice as long as the width of your hips.
❑ True
❑ False

7 – A good way to test the strength of a front stance is by exerting pressure on the rear of the back leg knee, and by pushing the hips toward the rear.
❑ True
❑ False

Notes:

8 – Front stance is considered an inside tension stance.
❑ True
❑ False

9 – Turning the front foot out away from the body center is not the correct position of the front foot in a front stance.
❑ True
❑ False

Notes:

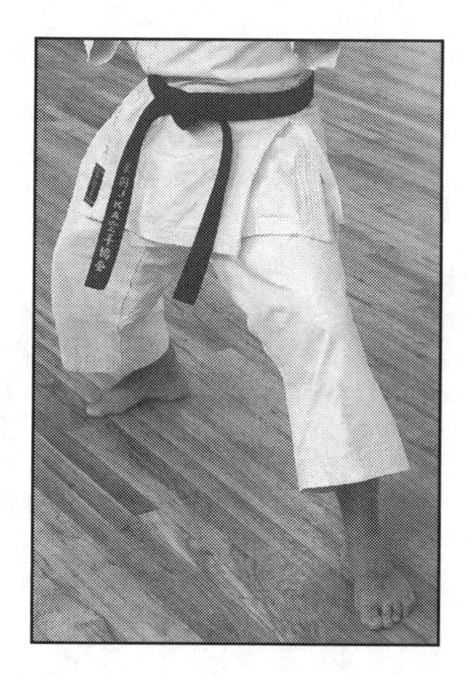

Back Stance–Key Points

Back stance is an outside tension stance with most of the weight, or "pressure", on the back leg–approximately 70% of the weight is on the back leg. The structure of the *back stance* is:

- the feet start at right angles to each other, and the feet form an "L" shape
- the back leg drops (steps) back to twice the width of the hips
- the front foot points forward, the back foot points to a right angle; maintain the "L" shape after dropping (stepping) back twice the width of the hips
- specifically, the little toes of both feet form the right angle to each other allowing the big toes to point slightly toward the body center

Insight to Kick Around

Back stance can be used to distance you from an opponent and allows the front leg to be "light" and ready to use for kicking.

Notes:

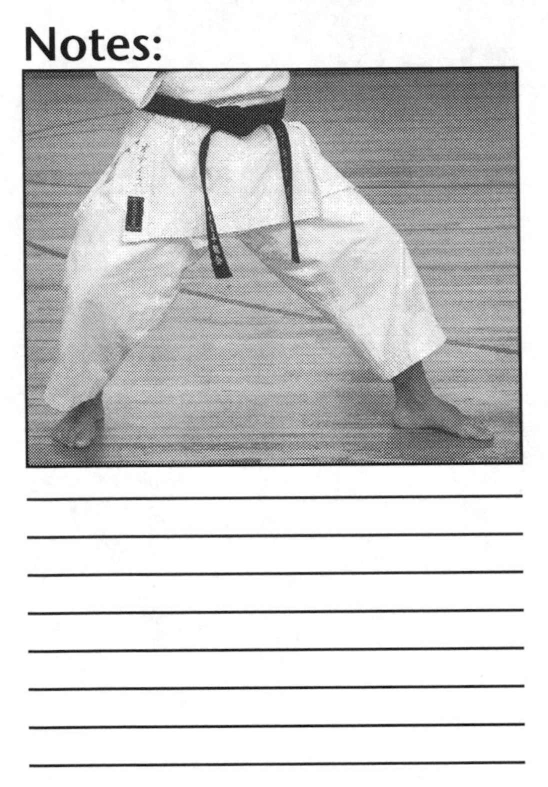

- the weight is down and the posture is straight and "correct"
- the knees are twisted out, and push away from each other, forming outside tension in the legs
- weight distribution is crucial–70% pressure on the rear leg

One of the purposes of a *back stance* is to separate or distance you from an opponent. The most fundamental point is the feeling that the front foot is actually pushing back, away from an opponent, adding extra pressure, or the correct 70% pressure, onto the back leg.

Common Errors

Common errors associated with *back stance:*

1- the length of the stance is either too short or too long, hindering movement and the strength of the stance

2- the front foot position should not be turned in or out
  - the hip, front knee, and front foot toe form a straight line

3- the hip position should not be twisted out
  - the hip position is not tucking beneath the torso,which causes the face and upper body to bend forward, making it impossible to respond to an attack

Training Method for Back Stance

To check the effectiveness and correctness of a *back stance,* it is important to test three areas: the distribution of weight, the ability to use the front leg for kicking, and posture so the face remains away from an attack.

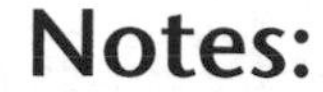

To Test the Strength of a Back Stance

1- assume a *back stance*

2- have someone stand in front of you, place their hands on your hips, and push towards the rear
   - you should not fall or lose the structure of the "L" shape *back stance*

To Test Posture While in Back Stance

1- assume a *back stance*

2- have someone stand to your side and run a hand in a straight line, starting on top of the head (but in front of the face) to the base of the hips
   - if the posture is wrong, the hand will run into the head/face, chest, or stomach.
   - it is crucial that the nose, chest, and stomach are in a straight line

To Test the Ability to Use the Front Leg for Kicking While in Back Stance

1- assume a *back stance*

2- have someone stand to your side and place a hand in front of your chest

3- while in *back stance*, raise the front knee toward the chest
   - the front knee and leg should raise smoothly without drastically changing the distribution of weight onto the back leg (it should retain approximately 70% of the body weight/pressure of the stance)
   - posture should remain intact; the head does not lean forward nor should the hips move back away from the torso

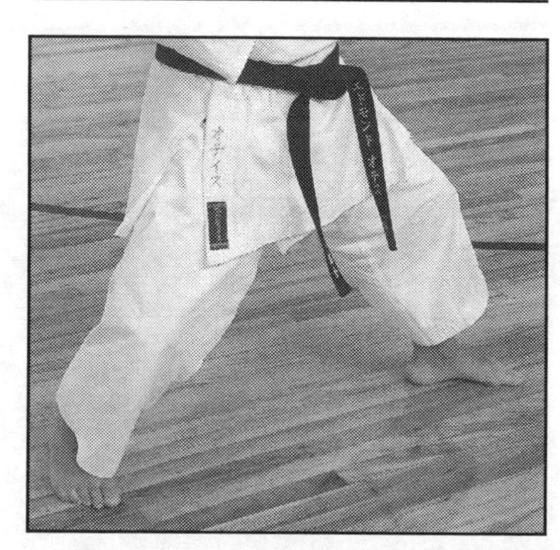

Notes:

Close Up and Review

View the close up and review in the Back Stance section of the Essential Shotokan DVD or VHS tape.

NOTE:

The back stance *smoothly* pushes away using the front leg, causing the rear leg to sustain approximately 70% of the body weight/pressure. Correct posture keeps the face distant from a potential facial attack–even while stepping/dropping back onto the rear leg–and provides a natural, relaxed stance. *Both* knees bend in a back stance; the front leg knee of a back stance slightly bends.

Stance in Action

Watch *back stance* "in action" on the Essential Shotokan DVD or VHS tape.

NOTE:

A properly executed *back stance* separates the face and torso from an advancing attack and allows seamless use of the front leg for kicking.

Notes:

Q and A

1 – Back stance has absolutely nothing in common with posture.
❑ True
❑ False

2 – Approximately 30% of the overall body weight distribution is on the front leg of a back stance.
❑ True
❑ False

3 – The feet are at right angles to each other.
❑ True
❑ False

4 – The hip, front leg knee, and front foot big toe form a straight line.
❑ True
❑ False

5 – If posture is correct in a back stance, you will intersect the top of the head when running your hand in front of the body in a downward motion.
❑ True
❑ False

6 – The front foot should never twist in or away from the body center.
❑ True
❑ False

7 – Only the back knee is bent in back stance.
❑ True
❑ False

Notes:

8 – The front foot has the feeling of pushing toward the rear in a back stance.
❑ True
❑ False

9 – The right angle, or "L" shape, of a back stance is formed using the little toes of both feet as the outer edge of the stance.
❑ True
❑ False

Hour Glass Stance Key Points

Notes:

Hour glass stance is one of the first fundamental inside tension stances used in Shotokan karate. This type of inside tension stance positions the width of the feet about as wide as the hips. In order to make strength, it is important to lower the hips (bend the knees) and twist both knees in toward the body center.

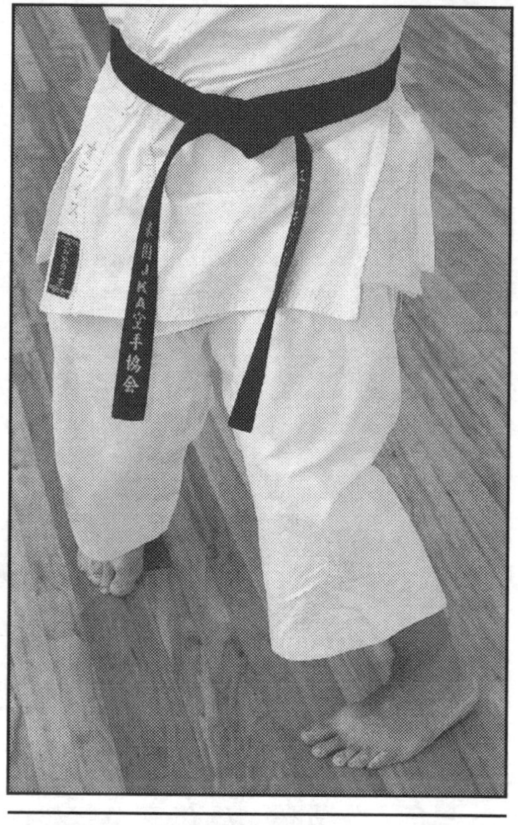

The Hour Glass Stance Structure

- step forward so the front foot heel is in line with the rear foot toes
- the heel of the front foot forms a straight, horizontal line to the toes of the rear foot
- position the feet only as wide as the hips
- the rear foot points "straight" forward
- the front foot is turned in at about a 45° angle
- maintain a natural "correct" posture from the top of the head to the tailbone
- tuck the hips underneath the torso
- collapse the legs (knees) inside (toward the body center), squeezing the inside of the thighs together (inward)

Common Errors

Common errors associated with *hour glass stance* mostly have to do with posture, foot position, and leg tension.

1-feet position: make sure the stance is not too long or too short, only hip-width

Insight to Kick Around
Hour glass stance is an inside tension stance that is typically used "in-close" to an opponent.

Notes:

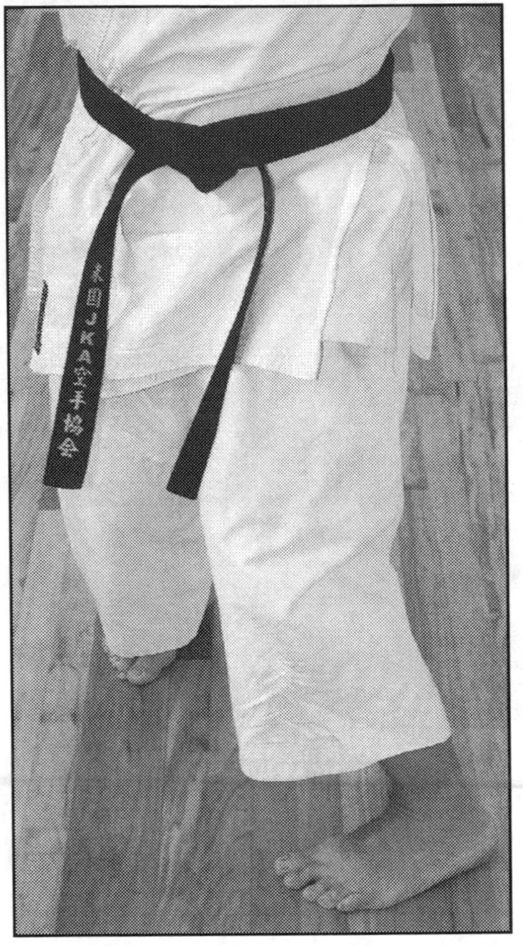

2- posture: make sure the hips are not tucked *too far* forward or sticking out to the rear

3- inside leg tension–it is crucial that the legs squeeze together strongly

4- make sure there is no gap between the legs, but that the thighs press (squeeze) together–both knees press to the body center

Training Method for Hour Glass Stance

Hour glass stance (as well as other inside tension stances) is usually used if you're close to an opponent. In this type of stance/ position it is crucial to lower the body center to make a strong position, even though your feet are close together.

Listed Below Are Three Hour Glass Stance Training Methods

1 - Lifting the *hour glass stance:*

- assume an *hour glass stance*
- have someone stand behind you and attempt to lift you up

NOTE: If your hips are lowered, if the posture is correct, and there is proper tension in the legs, you should feel very *heavy and dense* and not be easy to lift up.

Variation–Dropping Into Hour Glass Stance

2 - Assume the proper feet positions for *hour glass stance* but *do not* lower the hips or squeeze the legs together:

- have someone stand behind you and wrap their arms around your torso at chest level

Notes:

- as the person with the hands wrapped around your body attempts to lift, quickly assume a full *hour glass stance*
- drop the hips, bend the knees toward the body center, and squeeze the thighs together, causing the *hour glass stance* to become heavy and dense, pulling the person behind you downward
- maintain proper posture throughout

3 - Kicking toward the groin in *hour glass stance:*

NOTE: *Even though you may be close to an opponent, by holding the knees in an inside position, you're able to protect the groin. Test this by simply kicking toward the groin, carefully!*

- assume an *hour glass stance*
- at a close distance, have someone kick lightly toward the groin
- if the knees are not close together, the kicking leg will easily rise up and hit the groin

  SAFETY NOTE: Please simulate hitting the groin when practicing this training method of *hour glass stance.* Never hit your training partner in the groin!

- bring the knees inward toward each other (toward the body center) to avoid injury by preventing the kicking leg from reaching the groin, and *simultaneously* maintain correct

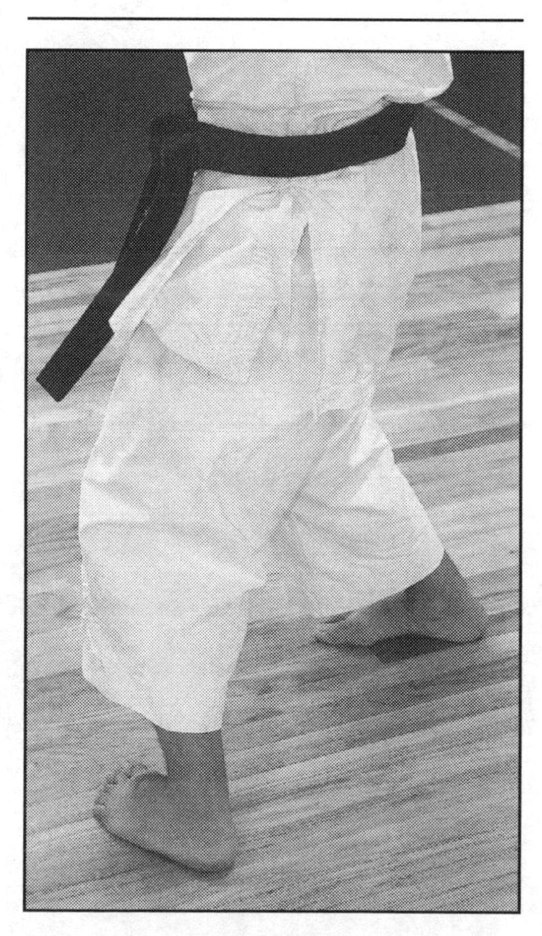

Notes:

posture, lower the hips, and squeeze the thighs together, causing the *hour glass stance* to become heavy and dense

Close Up and Review

View the close up and review in the Hour Glass Stance section of the Essential Shotokan DVD or VHS tape.

NOTE:

The *hour glass stance* is a dense and heavy inside tension stance that maintains proper posture and protects the groin region at close distances.

Q and A

1 – Hour glass stance has no concerns regarding posture.
❑ True
❑ False

2 – Hour glass stance is an outside tension stance.
❑ True
❑ False

3 – It should be easy to lift someone from behind in an hour glass stance.
❑ True
❑ False

4 – The feet are twice the width of the hips in hour glass stance.
❑ True
❑ False

Notes:

5 – The back foot points at a 45° angle in hour glass stance.
- ❑ True
- ❑ False

6 – The hips lowered, the thighs and knees squeezed together, and correct posture work together to make an hour glass stance heavy and dense.
- ❑ True
- ❑ False

7 – Protecting the groin at close distance is one feature of hour glass stance.
- ❑ True
- ❑ False

Notes:

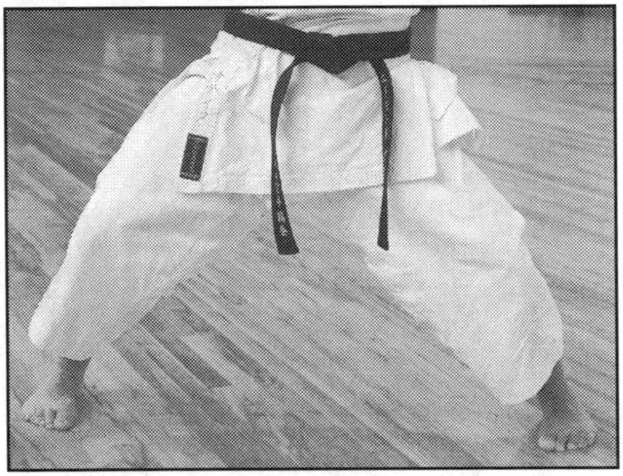

Side Stance–Key Points

Side Stance or *horse stance* is an outside tension stance and has two purposes in Shotokan karate. First, as a training stance, *side stance* is used to develop strength in the hips and legs while practicing upper body techniques. Additionally, *side stance* is used offensively or defensively to the sides.

The Structure of a Side Stance

- the stance is about two hip-widths wide *Note:* Side stance is the same width as the length of front stance and back stance.
- the weight of the stance is equally distributed between both legs
- both feet are pointed forward
- the little toe of each foot points forward so the big toes of each foot point in slightly
- the posture is natural and "correct"– the tailbone tucks underneath the torso
- most importantly, twist (torque) the knees outward against the stance (away from the

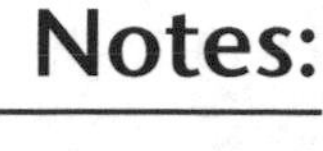

body center, creating outside tension in the legs) which brings strength and tightness to the body center

- at all times the body sits "in stance" in a relaxed manner

Common Errors

Common errors associated with *side stance:*

1- allowing the feet to twist outward
  - prevents the possibility of outside tension in the stance

2- allowing the hips to push outside (to the rear) or unnaturally underneath the torso
  - prevents the natural contraction of the muscles or natural use of the stance; make sure the posture is straight all the way from the tail bone to the top of the head

3- raising the shoulders up
  - prevents (hinders) tensing and use of the body center

Training Method for Side Stance

To test the strength of a *side stance* (or *horse stance*), we will take a look at two dimensions of the stance:

1- the ability to keep the weight down in *side stance*

2- the ability to support the weight of the stance itself

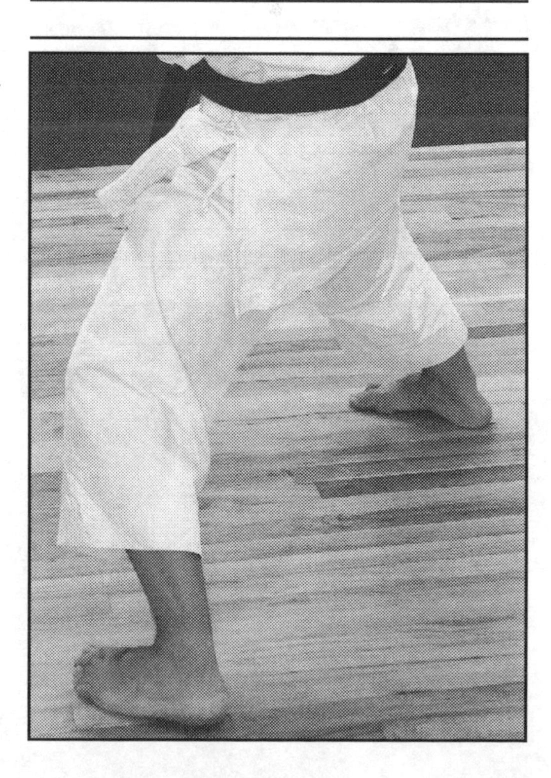

Notes:

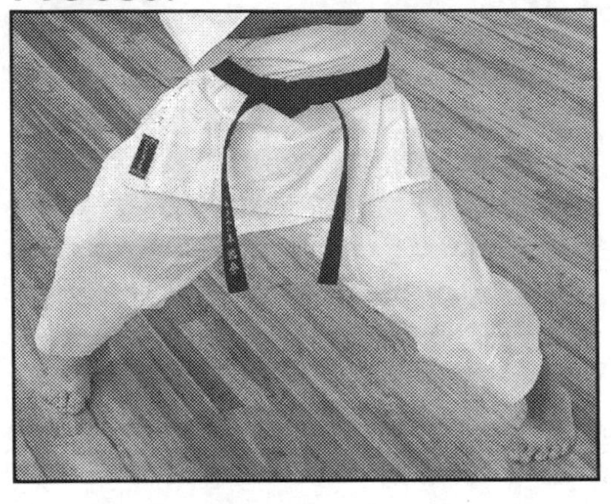

To Test the Ability to Keep the Weight Down in Side Stance

- assume a *side stance*
- have someone stand behind you and attempt to lift you out of the stance

  Note: If the body weight is down, it will be difficult to raise the body up from the side stance. If the body weight is not down, it will be simple to raise the body up out of the side stance.

To Test the Ability to Support the Weight of the Stance Itself

- assume a *side stance*
- have someone stand behind you and apply weight to the stance with downward pressure by leaning their body weight on your shoulders

  Note: This will force the stance to not only support you, but to also support the weight of the person applying the downward pressure.

Close Up and Review

View the close up and review in the Side Stance section of the Essential Shotokan DVD or VHS tape.

NOTE:

Carefully note, while the *side stance* steps out approximately two times the width of the hips, the action of the body center is to *drop while stepping* into the stance. You should not step out two hip widths first, then drop into side stance; rather, you should *begin* the stance by dropping the body center (torso)–maintain the proper alignment of posture–*while* stepping out into side stance.

Notes:

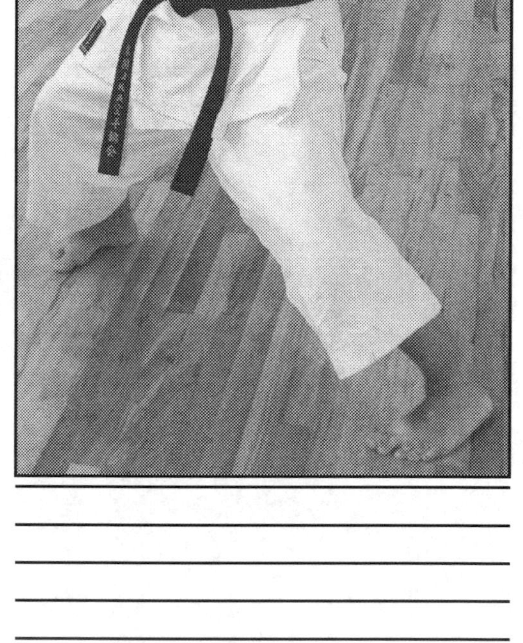

Stance in Action

Watch *side stance* "in action" on the Essential Shotokan DVD or VHS tape.

NOTE:

All the defensive techniques executed from *side stance* occur from a *deeply* set stance. Additionally, all the *side stances* used "in action" *begin* by lowering the body center *before setting* the stance to block or strike; the block, strike, and side stance all come together at the point of focus.

Q and A

1 – Side stance has no concerns regarding posture.
❑ True
❑ False

2 – Side stance is only as wide as your hips.
❑ True
❑ False

3 – Your hips should push away, toward the rear, in a side stance.
❑ True
❑ False

4 – Keep your little toes pointing out at 45° from the body center for a stable side stance.
❑ True
❑ False

5 – The side stance is an inside tension stance.
❑ True
❑ False

Notes:

6 – The position of the knees in side stance should push away from the body center to assist in outside tension.
❑ True
❑ False

7 – The body weight in side stance applies downward pressure.
❑ True
❑ False

Bonus Question

1 – Studying body dynamics and stances is extremely important to Shotokan karate.
❑ True
❑ False

Final Note From the Authors

We know that the bonus question is simplistic, but our intent is to convey how much we believe the principles and stances presented in this volume of the Essential Shotokan series are not optional; they are fundamentally necessary.

Notes:

Notes:

Chapter 5: Q and A Answers

Notes:

Chapter 1: Introduction

Introduction Q and A, Page 2

1 – The Essential Shotokan series is designed only for advanced karate students.
- ❑ True
- ■ False

2 – The relationship between core principles and technique makes the study of Shotokan unique.
- ■ True
- ❑ False

3 – The ultimate goal in training in karate is to handle a conflict with violence.
- ❑ True
- ■ False

4 – Should karate training develop a level of technical and emotional mastery to be used when an opponent is at their weakest?
- ■ Yes
- ❑ No

Notes:

Chapter 3: Focus

Focus Q and A, Pages 7-8

1 – Focus is by far not one of the most essential aspects of Shotokan karate.
❑ True
■ False

2 – Focus is a coordination of body reaction, body action, breathing, and technique.
■ True
❑ False

3 – A simple formula for focus can be thought of as:
❑ To focus, generate as much force as possible, over the longest period of time, into the largest impact area.
■ To focus, generate as much force as possible, over the shortest period of time, into the smallest impact area.

4 – Concerning focus, two things are important:
❑ To focus, combine speed and the overall quality of the technique.
■ Combine range and body actions with breathing.

Notes:

5 – It can be said:
- ❑ Moving quickly from one technique to another without interruption will improve the range of focus.
- ■ One method employed to train a soft movement, to then be compressed at the end of a movement (technique) as an aspect of focus and range, is by holding the end of the technique.

6 – Coordinating body actions with breating is not as important as muscular strength.
- ❑ True
- ■ False

Posture Q and A, Page 11

1 – Correct posture allows us to:
- ❑ relax and sleep
- ■ move, set, and wait with poise so we can react

2 – One of the six key principles of correct posture is:
- ❑ Keep the body tense at all times.
- ■ Keep the shoulders down, resting on the body, with no tension.

3 – For correct posture, the body weight position should allow for the heels to be off the floor at all times.
- ❑ True
- ■ False

Notes:

Six Body Actions Q and A, Page 13

1 – Which is not a body action?
- ■ muscular strength
- ❑ pendulum action

2 – Pendulum action is primarily used in blocking.
- ❑ True
- ■ False

3 – Body shifting is done by rotation of the hips.
- ❑ True
- ■ False

4 – Of all the body actions, vibration is the slowest and least immediate.
- ❑ True
- ■ False

Vibration Q and A, page 15

1 – In body vibration, less emphasis is placed on the hip and more is placed on the arm.
- ❑ True
- ■ False

2 – Momentum does not play a role in body vibration.
- ❑ True
- ■ False

3 – Body vibration works best with a slow hip snap.
- ❑ True
- ■ False

Notes:

Body/hip Rotation Q and A, Page 17

1 – Body/hip rotation is not used in anything other than karate techniques.
❑ True
■ False

2 – Reverse reaction rotation is a type of body/hip rotation.
■ True
❑ False

3 – Body/hip rotation only rotates the hips, leaving the upper part of the torso unmoved.
❑ True
■ False

4 – A key point in the rotation principle is the similarity to swinging the body with a bat in your hands to hit a baseball.
■ True
❑ False

Body Shifting Q and A, Page 19

1 – Body shifting creates power by keeping the body still; momentum is not needed.
❑ True
■ False

2 – An example of body shifting is displacing another person's stance by bumping into them.
■ True
❑ False

Notes:

3 – Stepping or sliding the body forward, back, left, or right are both methods of body shifting.
■ True
❑ False

4 – Body shifting generates power and momentum for striking and punching.
■ True
❑ False

Body Dropping Q and A, Page 21

1 – Chopping wood utilizes the principle of body dropping.
■ True
❑ False

2 – Pushing the body center away from the target and bending fully at the waist is a correct description of the body action known as *body dropping*.
❑ True
■ False

3 – You should not bend your knees when attempting the body dropping principle.
❑ True
■ False

4 – It is best to inhale when using the body dropping principle.
❑ True
■ False

Body Raising/Lifting Q and A, Page 23

1 – Body lifting is best done with the muscles of the back.
- ❑ True
- ■ False

2 – Body lifting drives the body from a low position up into the attack.
- ■ True
- ❑ False

3 – A good example of body lifting is:
- ❑ keep the knees straight, and bend at the waist to pick up an object from the floor
- ■ squat down low to the ground, and drive up (raise up) the body using the legs (muscles)

4 – It is best to hold your breath when using the principle of lift weight.
- ❑ True
- ■ False

Pendulum Action Q and A, Page 25

1 – Pendulum action ideally is used when you are extremely far from your target.
- ❑ True
- ■ False

2 – Pendulum action is a small body action.
- ■ True
- ❑ False

Notes:

Notes:

3 – The central axis of the hips rotate in place during pendulum action.
■ True
❑ False

4 – Pendulum action drives the impact of the kicking foot or knee.
■ True
❑ False

Breathing Q and A, Page 27

1 – Breathing during a technique is *only* to prevent you from passing out.
❑ True
■ False

2 – What is most important in bringing the breathing and the technique together?
■ timing
❑ squeezing the muscles slowly

3 – Breathing (exhaling) plays a role in protecting me by helping to absorb an incoming technique at the point of impact.
■ True
❑ False

4 – *Heian nidan* teaches you to exhale once during every technique without multiple focal compressions.
❑ True
■ False

Notes:

5 – Two type of breathing have been discussed: First, one breath per technique; second, one breath with multiple techniques and multiple focal compressions.
■ True
❑ False

Timing Q and A, Pages 32 - 33

1 – The most fundamental way to think of timing has to do with addressing an opponent's attack.
■ True
❑ False

2 – Regarding the timing principle *after* (an opponent's attack), you respond with a counter attack after blocking.
■ True
❑ False

3 – Timing the movement to hit an opponent advancing toward you is called catching the opponent *during* the attack.
■ True
❑ False

4 – How much time you have to respond to an opponent plays a large role in what type of timing response you employ.
■ True
❑ False

Notes:

5 – Rhythm timing has to do with catching your opponent by surprise.
❑ True
■ False

6 – Reaction timing takes into account the movement of your opponent.
❑ True
■ False

7 – Use of an opponent's body movement and technique to set up a counter attack uses which timing principle?
■ rhythm timing
❑ reaction timing

8 – Catching an opponent by surprise or standing still employs which timing principle?
❑ rhythm timing
■ reaction timing

9 – If an opponent escapes at the same time, moves the same distance, and travels at the same speed as the attacker, there is very little chance of the attacker catching the opponent.
■ True
❑ False

Notes:

Chapter 4: Stances

Natural/Yoi Stance Q and A, Page 38

1 – Natural stance, ready stance, and *yoi* position is *Hachiji Tachi.*
■ True
❑ False

2 – Posture is only important to natural stance when performing kata.
❑ True
■ False

3 – For a good *yoi* position, tighten all your muscles tightly so you can focus your concentration.
❑ True
■ False

4 – If *yoi* position is done correctly, my opponent will not know I am ready to engage in sparring.
■ True
❑ False

5 – The command, "*Yoi*," literally means *ready position.*
❑ True
■ False

6 – Natural/ready/*yoi* stance coordinates concentration of mind and body.
■ True
❑ False

Notes:

Free Stance Q and A, Pages 40 - 41

1 – Free stance has absolutely nothing in common with natural stance.
❑ True
■ False

2 – Free stance can be used to engage in a conflict or combative role.
■ True
❑ False

3 – Free stance is just as long as a forward stance.
❑ True
■ False

4 – Free stance should have the body weight totally committed to the front or to the rear but never smoothly distributed between the legs.
❑ True
■ False

5 – Free stance generally places most of the weight on the balls of the feet.
■ True
❑ False

6 – Tucking the hips underneath the torso tightens the lower body and does not allow the body to move smoothly to the front, side, and back.
❑ True
■ False

7 – Tension in the upper or lower body will prevent a *karateka* from moving in free stance effectively.
■ True
❑ False

Notes:

Front Stance Q and A, Pages 45 - 46

1 – Front stance has absolutely nothing in common with posture.
- ❑ True
- ■ False

2 – Front stance places most of the weight on the back foot.
- ❑ True
- ■ False

3 – The hips should be driven forward by the heel and extension of the back leg in a front stance.
- ■ True
- ❑ False

4 – The driving force of the back leg starts on the balls of the feet.
- ❑ True
- ■ False

5 – The width of a front stance is as wide as your hips.
- ■ True
- ❑ False

6 – The length of a front stance is about twice as long as the width of your hips.
- ■ True
- ❑ False

7 – A good way to test the strength of a front stance is by exerting pressure on the rear of the back leg knee, and by pushing the hips toward the rear.
- ■ True
- ❑ False

Notes:

8 – Front stance is considered an inside tension stance.
- ❑ True
- ■ False

9 – Turning the front foot out away from the body center is not the correct position of the front foot in a front stance.
- ■ True
- ❑ False

Back Stance Q and A, Pages 51 - 52

1 – Back stance has absolutely nothing in common with posture.
- ❑ True
- ■ False

2 – Approximately 30% of the overall body weight distribution is on the front leg of a back stance.
- ■ True
- ❑ False

3 – The back stance feet positions are at right angles to each other.
- ■ True
- ❑ False

4 – The hip, front leg knee, and front foot big toe form a straight line in back stance.
- ■ True
- ❑ False

Notes:

5 – If posture is correct in a back stance you will intersect the top of the head when running your hand in front of the body in a downward motion.
❑ True
■ False

6 – The front foot should never twist in or away from the body center.
■ True
❑ False

7 – Only the back knee is bent in back stance.
❑ True
■ False

8 – The front foot has the feeling of pushing toward the rear in a back stance.
■ True
❑ False

9 – The right angle, or "L" shape, of a back stance is formed using the little toes of both feet as the outer edge of the stance.
■ True
❑ False

Hour Glass Q and A, Page 56 - 57

1 – Hour glass stance has no concerns regarding posture.
❑ True
■ False

2 – Hour glass stance is an outside tension stance.
❑ True
■ False

Notes:

3 – It should be easy to lift someone from behind in an hour glass stance.
❑ True
■ False

4 – The feet are twice the width of the hips in hour glass stance.
❑ True
■ False

5 – The back foot points at a 45° angle in hour glass stance.
❑ True
■ False

6 – The hips lowered, the thighs and knees squeezed together, and correct posture work together to make an hour glass stance heavy and dense.
■ True
❑ False

7 – Protecting the groin at close distance is one feature of hour glass stance.
■ True
❑ False

Side Stance Q and A, Pages 61 - 62

1 – Side stance has no concerns regarding posture.
❑ True
■ False

2 – Side stance is only as wide as your hips.
❑ True
■ False

Notes:

3 – Your hips should push away, toward the rear, in a side stance.
❑ True
■ False

4 – Keep your little toes pointing out at 45° from the body center for a stable side stance.
❑ True
■ False

5 – The side stance is an inside tension stance.
❑ True
■ False

6 – The position of the knees in side stance should push away from the body center to assist in outside tension.
■ True
❑ False

7 – The body weight in side stance applies downward pressure.
■ True
❑ False

Bonus Question:

1 – Studying body dynamics and stances is extremely important to Shotokan karate.
■ True
❑ False